HEALING PANCREATITIS

A Comprehensive Guide to the Pancreatitis Diet

Dr Philip Ortner

TABLE OF CONTENTS

CHAPTER 1

Understanding Pancreatitis

Pancreatitis is a condition that affects the pancreas, a vital organ tucked away behind your stomach. To understand this ailment, we need to unravel its intricacies, starting with what pancreatitis is, the different types it comes in, what sets it off, and how it shows itself.

Definition and Types of Pancreatitis

At its core, pancreatitis is the inflammation of the pancreas. Now, the pancreas is not just a random organ; it plays a pivotal role in our digestive system and helps regulate blood sugar. Imagine it as a multitasking wizard behind the scenes. When something goes wrong and the pancreas becomes inflamed, that's pancreatitis.

There are two main types of pancreatitis: acute and chronic. Acute pancreatitis is like a sudden storm – it hits hard and fast. It's often caused by gallstones or excessive alcohol consumption, two factors that can irritate the pancreas. Chronic pancreatitis, on the other hand, is more like a persistent drizzle. It develops over time, and while it shares some causes with acute pancreatitis, it's often linked to long-term alcohol abuse or certain medical conditions.

Causes and Risk Factors:

Pancreatitis doesn't just happen out of the blue; there are usually reasons behind it. Gallstones are a common culprit for acute pancreatitis. These small, hard particles can block the pancreatic duct, triggering inflammation. Excessive alcohol consumption is another significant player. The pancreas doesn't appreciate being bombarded with alcohol, and over time, this can lead to chronic pancreatitis.

But it's not just about gallstones and alcohol. Sometimes, certain infections, trauma to the abdomen, or even high levels of fats in the blood can set off pancreatitis. There's also a sneaky condition called hereditary pancreatitis, where a genetic factor makes some individuals more prone to developing pancreatitis.

Now, let's talk about risk factors. These are the elements that increase your chances of getting pancreatitis. Obesity is one of them. Extra weight, especially around the abdomen, can apply pressure on the pancreas and contribute to inflammation. High levels of triglycerides, a type of fat in the blood, can also up the risk. Certain medications, smoking, and even a family history of pancreatitis can make you more susceptible.

Symptoms and Diagnosis

Pancreatitis comes with its own set of signals, like a desperate cry for attention from your pancreas. The symptoms can range from mildly annoying to downright excruciating. Picture this: severe pain in the upper abdomen that may radiate to your back – that's a classic symptom. It's the kind of pain that demands attention, often requiring a visit to the emergency room.

Nausea and vomiting often accompany the pain, as the digestive system rebels against the inflamed pancreas. You might notice your abdomen becoming tender to the touch, and your body might throw in a fever just to keep things interesting.

Now, diagnosing pancreatitis involves a combination of your medical history, a physical examination, and some tests. Blood tests can reveal higher levels of pancreatic enzymes, a telltale sign of pancreatitis. Imaging tests, like CT scans or MRIs, can give a closer look at the pancreas and identify any abnormalities. Sometimes, an endoscopic ultrasound might be needed to get an even more detailed view.

Understanding pancreatitis means recognizing the signs and symptoms early on. If you experience persistent abdominal pain, especially coupled with vomiting and nausea, it's time to seek medical attention. Early detection can make a significant difference in managing pancreatitis effectively.

CHAPTER 2

The Importance of Diet in Pancreatitis Management

Welcome to the nutritional battleground where the choices we make with our forks can either calm the storm or add fuel to the fire. In this chapter, we'll explore how diet plays a crucial role in managing pancreatitis, why what you eat matters, and how making the right food choices can be a game-changer in preventing those painful flare-ups. But first, let's understand how the battleground is set – how diet impacts the health of our pancreas.

How Diet Impacts Pancreatic Health

Imagine your pancreas as a delicate instrument, finely tuned to handle the digestive orchestra in your body. When it's healthy, it secretes enzymes that help break down food so your body can absorb the nutrients. Now, when inflammation hits (hello, pancreatitis!), this delicate balance is disrupted.

Certain foods can either soothe or irritate the already inflamed pancreas. Think of it like pouring lemon juice on a paper cut – not the best idea. That's why understanding how diet impacts pancreatic health is crucial. It's not just about avoiding the bad stuff; it's also about embracing the good stuff that can aid in the healing process.

Role of Nutrition in Preventing Flare-Ups

Picture your pancreas as a superhero, and nutrition is its sidekick. Proper nutrition can be the Robin to your pancreas' Batman, helping to prevent flare-ups and keeping the bad guys (inflammation) at bay. So, what does this dynamic duo look like in terms of food?

First and foremost, it's about maintaining a balanced diet. This means getting the right mix of proteins, carbohydrates, fats, vitamins, and minerals. Proteins are like the construction workers, helping repair and build tissues. Carbohydrates are the energy providers, keeping everything running smoothly. Fats play a role too, but it's about choosing the right kinds – the unsaturated fats that won't aggravate your pancreas.

Fiber is another essential player. It's like the broom that sweeps away the debris in your digestive system, ensuring everything moves along without causing trouble. And let's not forget hydration. Water is the lubricant that keeps the gears turning, helping your pancreas do its job more efficiently.

Now, there's a superhero diet called the low-fat diet. This is like putting your pancreas on a spa day. Since too much fat can be a trigger for pancreatitis, a low-fat diet is often recommended to keep things in check. Lean proteins, fruits, vegetables, and whole grains become your trusty sidekicks in this dietary adventure.

But it's not just about what you eat; it's also about how you eat. Small, frequent meals are the strategy here. Instead of bombarding your pancreas with a massive feast, spreading your meals throughout the day puts less stress on your digestive system. It's like giving your pancreas mini-missions rather than an all-out war.

Common Dietary Mistakes to Avoid

Now, let's talk about the pitfalls – the dietary mistakes that can turn your nutritional ally into a formidable foe. One major slip-up is overindulging in fatty foods. Remember, too much fat can be like throwing gasoline on the inflammation fire. So, it's crucial to be mindful of your fat intake and opt for healthier fats like those found in avocados, nuts, and olive oil.

Alcohol is another antagonist in the pancreatitis saga. It's like handing your pancreas a Molotov cocktail. The inflammation caused by alcohol can be a significant trigger for pancreatitis or worsen an existing condition. So, if you're serious about managing pancreatitis, limiting or eliminating alcohol is a non-negotiable.

Skipping meals is a third misstep. It's like sending your pancreas into battle without armor. When you skip meals, your pancreas is left to deal with a sudden influx of food when you finally decide to eat. This can strain an already compromised system, leading to more discomfort and potential flare-ups.

Processed foods are the stealthy enemies in this dietary war. Packed with additives, preservatives, and unhealthy fats, they can wreak havoc on your pancreas. Opting for whole, unprocessed foods is like giving your pancreas a breath of fresh air – it can focus on digesting nutrients rather than battling unnecessary chemicals.

In this chapter, we've embarked on a journey into the heart of nutritional management for pancreatitis. We've explored how diet impacts the delicate balance of the pancreas, the superheroic role of nutrition in preventing flare-ups, and the common dietary mistakes that can sabotage your efforts. Armed with this knowledge, you're now better equipped to navigate the dietary maze and make choices that support, rather than hinder, your pancreas on its path to recovery.

CHAPTER 3

Building a Foundation Pancreatitis-Friendly Foods

Welcome to the heart of healing, where we explore the foods that can be your pancreas's best friends. In this chapter, we'll take a closer look at the superheroes of the pantry – the foods that not only support pancreatic health but also contribute to an overall sense of well-being. So, let's dive into the world of pancreatitis-friendly foods.

Overview of Foods that Support Pancreatic Health

Think of your pancreas as a delicate garden that needs just the right nutrients to bloom. Pancreatitis-friendly foods are like the nourishing soil, the sunlight, and the rain that help your pancreatic garden flourish. So, what are these magical foods?

1. Lean Proteins: Proteins are the building blocks of life, and for your pancreas, they're the construction workers helping in the repair and regeneration process. Opt for lean proteins like chicken, turkey, fish, and tofu. These proteins provide the necessary amino acids without the excess fat that could trigger inflammation.

2. Fruits and Vegetables: Imagine a burst of color on your plate – that's the vibrant array of fruits and vegetables. These powerhouses are rich in vitamins, minerals, and antioxidants. They're like the defenders of your pancreatic fortress, helping to reduce inflammation and support the healing process. Think berries, citrus fruits, leafy greens, and colorful veggies.

3. Whole Grains: Carbohydrates are your body's primary energy source, and whole grains are the gold standard. They release energy slowly, keeping your blood sugar levels stable. Foods like brown rice, quinoa, oats, and whole wheat bread are the unsung heroes of your pancreas, providing sustained energy without causing unnecessary stress.

4. Healthy Fats: Not all fats are villains; some can be heroes too. Healthy fats, like those found in avocados, nuts, seeds, and olive oil, are like the guardians of balance. They provide essential fatty acids without overloading your pancreas, ensuring a smooth and harmonious digestion process.

5. Dairy or Dairy Alternatives: Calcium is crucial for your bones and overall health, and dairy or fortified dairy alternatives can be a good source. Opt for low-fat or fat-free options to keep your fat intake in check. Milk, yogurt, and plant-based alternatives like almond or soy milk can be part of a pancreatitis-friendly diet.

The Significance of a Well-Balanced Diet

Now that we've met our pancreatitis-friendly superheroes, let's understand the importance of assembling them into a well-balanced diet. Think of a balanced diet as the conductor of a symphony. Each instrument (food group) has a role to play, and when they harmonize, the result is a masterpiece – in this case, optimal pancreatic health.

1. Providing Essential Nutrients: A well-balanced diet ensures that your body, and specifically your pancreas, gets all the essential nutrients it needs. Proteins for repair, carbohydrates for energy, fats for cell structure, vitamins for overall health – it's like a nutrient orchestra working in sync.

2. Maintaining Blood Sugar Levels: Stability is the key when it comes to blood sugar levels.

Whole grains and complex carbohydrates release energy gradually, preventing spikes and crashes in blood sugar. This stability is essential for managing pancreatitis and reducing stress on your pancreas.

3. Supporting Digestive Health: The digestive system is a complex network, and a well-balanced diet keeps everything moving smoothly. Fiber from fruits, vegetables, and whole grains acts like a broom, sweeping away debris and promoting regular bowel movements. This is crucial for preventing complications and discomfort associated with pancreatitis.

4. Reducing Inflammation: Inflammation is the enemy in pancreatitis, and certain foods have anti-inflammatory properties. Fruits, vegetables, and foods rich in omega-3 fatty acids (like fatty fish) can help keep inflammation at bay. It's like having a team of firefighters ready to extinguish any inflammatory sparks.

Nutrient-Rich Options for Optimal Recovery

Now, let's explore specific nutrient-rich options that can take your pancreatitis-friendly diet to the next level, promoting optimal recovery and overall well-being.

1. Omega-3 Fatty Acids: Fatty fish, such as salmon, mackerel, and sardines, are rich in omega-3 fatty acids. These fats have anti-inflammatory properties and can contribute to the healing process. Consider incorporating fish into your diet a couple of times a week.

2. Antioxidant-Rich Foods: Antioxidants are like the superheroes that fight against oxidative stress in your body. Berries (blueberries, strawberries, raspberries), dark chocolate, and even green tea are packed with antioxidants. They help combat inflammation and support the recovery of your pancreas.

3. Probiotics: Probiotics are the friendly bacteria that support your gut health. Yogurt with live cultures, kefir, and fermented foods like sauerkraut can introduce these beneficial microbes into your system. A healthy gut contributes to overall well-being and may indirectly support your pancreas.

4. Hydration: Water is often underestimated, but it's a vital player in your recovery. Staying hydrated is like providing a refreshing drink to your pancreas, helping it function more efficiently. Aim for at least 8 glasses of water a day, more if you're physically active.

Putting It All Together: A Sample Pancreatitis-Friendly Meal

Let's create a culinary masterpiece that encompasses all these pancreatitis-friendly elements. How about a grilled salmon fillet (omega-3 fatty acids) with a side of quinoa (whole grains), a colorful salad of mixed berries and leafy greens (antioxidants), and a serving of plain yogurt (probiotics)? It's a symphony of flavors that not only satisfies your taste buds but also nourishes your pancreas.

CHAPTER 4

The Pancreatitis Diet: What to Eat

Welcome to the heart of your culinary journey towards a healthier pancreas. In this chapter, we'll delve into the specifics of the pancreatitis diet – the foods that can soothe rather than exacerbate, meal planning strategies tailored for individuals with pancreatitis, and some kitchen wizardry with recipes and cooking tips for a pancreatitis-friendly experience.

Specific Foods to Include in the Diet:

The pancreatitis diet is like a carefully curated guest list for a party your pancreas is hosting. Let's introduce the VIPs – the foods that are not only welcome but are essential for a harmonious digestive gathering.

1. Lean Proteins: Imagine a plate where the star is a grilled chicken breast or a piece of turkey. Lean proteins are the headliners of the pancreatitis diet. They provide the necessary amino acids for repair without burdening your pancreas with excessive fat. Fish, tofu, and legumes are also excellent choices in this category.

2. Fruits and Vegetables: This is the vibrant section of your plate, bursting with colors and nutrients. Berries, apples, carrots, spinach – the possibilities are endless. Fruits and vegetables are rich in vitamins, minerals, and antioxidants, supporting the healing process and reducing inflammation.

3. Whole Grains: Picture a side of quinoa or a serving of brown rice. Whole grains are like the reliable companions that provide sustained energy without causing undue stress on your pancreas. Oats, barley, and whole wheat products can be integral parts of your pancreatitis-friendly pantry.

4. Healthy Fats: Think of avocados, nuts, and olive oil as the wise counselors in your dietary kingdom. Healthy fats are essential for various bodily functions, and they can be included in moderation without triggering inflammation. These fats contribute to a well-rounded, pancreatitis-friendly diet.

5. Dairy or Dairy Alternatives: Calcium is crucial for bone health, and incorporating low-fat or fat-free dairy products or fortified dairy alternatives ensures you get this vital nutrient without overloading on fats. Yogurt, milk, and plant-based alternatives like almond or soy milk can be part of your daily intake.

6. Hydration: Water is the unsung hero of the pancreatitis diet. Staying well-hydrated is like providing a refreshing drink to your pancreas, helping it function more efficiently. Aim for at least 8 glasses of water a day, more if you're physically active.

Now, let's talk about how to orchestrate these ingredients into a well-balanced meal plan specifically tailored for individuals with pancreatitis.

Meal Planning for Individuals with Pancreatitis

Meal planning with pancreatitis involves more than just throwing ingredients together; it's about crafting a symphony of flavors that supports your digestive system. Here's a guide on how to structure your meals:

1. Small, Frequent Meals: Instead of three large meals, consider breaking your day into 5 or 6 smaller, balanced meals. This eases the digestive process for your pancreas, preventing it from being overwhelmed with a large influx of food.

2. Balanced Nutrients: Ensure that each meal includes a balance of proteins, carbohydrates, and healthy fats. This not only provides a comprehensive array of nutrients but also helps in stabilizing blood sugar levels and reducing the strain on your pancreas.

3. Snack Smart: Snacking can be an essential part of your meal plan. Opt for snacks that are nutrient-dense and easy on your pancreas. A handful of nuts, a piece of fruit, or some whole-grain crackers with hummus are excellent choices.

4. Limit or Avoid Trigger Foods: Identify and be mindful of foods that may trigger discomfort or worsen inflammation. For many, this includes high-fat foods, fried items, spicy dishes, and certain dairy products. Listen to your body and note any reactions to specific foods.

Recipes and Cooking Tips for a Pancreatitis-Friendly Kitchen

Now, let's bring the magic into the kitchen. Here are some recipes and cooking tips to turn your daily meals into a celebration of healing:

Recipe 1: Grilled Salmon with Lemon and Herbs:

- Ingredients:
    - Salmon fillets
    - Lemon juice
    - Fresh herbs (rosemary, thyme, or dill)
    - Olive oil
    - Salt and pepper to taste
- Instructions:

1. Preheat your grill or oven.
2. Place salmon fillets on a foil-lined baking sheet.

3. Drizzle with olive oil and lemon juice.

4. Sprinkle fresh herbs, salt, and pepper.

5. Grill or bake until the salmon is cooked through and flakes easily.

Recipe 2: Quinoa and Vegetable Stir-Fry:

- Ingredients:
    - Cooked quinoa
    - Mixed vegetables (bell peppers, broccoli, carrots)
    - Tofu or chicken (optional)
    - Low-sodium soy sauce
    - Garlic and ginger (minced)
    - Sesame oil
- Instructions:

    1. Stir-fry vegetables in sesame oil until slightly tender.

    2. Add tofu or chicken if desired.

    3. Mix in cooked quinoa.

    4. Add minced garlic and ginger.

5. Drizzle with low-sodium soy sauce and toss until well combined.

Cooking Tips

1. Steaming and Grilling: Opt for cooking methods like steaming and grilling instead of frying. These techniques preserve the nutritional value of foods without adding excessive fats.

2. Fresh Herbs and Spices: Use fresh herbs and spices to add flavor to your dishes without relying on excessive salt, sugar, or unhealthy fats. Experiment with basil, cilantro, mint, or a dash of turmeric for both taste and potential anti-inflammatory benefits.

3. Portion Control: Be mindful of portion sizes to avoid overeating. Smaller, frequent meals ensure a steady supply of nutrients without overwhelming your digestive system.

4. Food Diary: Consider keeping a food diary to track what you eat and how your body responds. This can help identify trigger foods or patterns that may be contributing to discomfort.

CHAPTER 5

Foods to Avoid: Triggers and Irritants

Welcome to the detective work of dietary management – identifying and eliminating the culprits that can exacerbate pancreatitis. In this chapter, we'll uncover the foods that can trigger discomfort, understand the impact of alcohol and caffeine on your pancreas, and navigate the delicate balance of limiting fat intake while making healthy fat choices.

Identifying and Eliminating Trigger Foods

Imagine your digestive system as a calm lake, and certain foods as rocks that create ripples of discomfort. Identifying and eliminating trigger foods is like removing those rocks, allowing the waters to settle. Here's how you can play detective to uncover your dietary culprits:

1. Keep a Food Diary: Start by keeping a detailed record of what you eat and how you feel afterward. Note any patterns of discomfort, bloating, or pain. This detective tool can help you identify specific foods that may be triggering your symptoms.

2. Monitor Portion Sizes: It's not just about what you eat; it's also about how much. Large portions, even of pancreatitis-friendly foods, can still cause discomfort. Pay attention to portion sizes and how your body responds to different quantities of food.

3. Gradual Elimination: If you suspect certain foods are causing issues, try eliminating them from your diet for a few weeks and observe any changes. Common triggers include spicy foods, high-fat items, and certain dairy products. Reintroduce one food at a time to pinpoint the troublemaker.

4. Pay Attention to Reactions: Listen to your body's signals. If you experience discomfort or notice changes in your digestive patterns after eating specific foods, take note. Your body is providing valuable clues about what agrees or disagrees with your pancreas.

Understanding the Impact of Alcohol and Caffeine

Now, let's talk about two common elements that can be double-edged swords when it comes to pancreatitis – alcohol and caffeine.

1. Alcohol: Alcohol is like a fiery dragon for your pancreas. It can be a significant trigger for pancreatitis or worsen an existing condition. When you consume alcohol, your pancreas has to work overtime to process it. This can lead to inflammation and irritation. For those with pancreatitis, it's often recommended to limit or completely eliminate alcohol from their diet.

Tips:

- If you choose to drink, do so in moderation, and always with food.
- Consider alternatives like non-alcoholic beer or mocktails to satisfy the social aspect without the alcohol content.

2. Caffeine: Caffeine is a stimulant that can have both positive and negative effects on your digestive system. While it can stimulate the release of digestive enzymes, too much caffeine can lead to increased stomach acid and irritation. It's like a jolt of energy for your pancreas, but an excessive jolt can cause more harm than good.

Tips:

- Monitor your caffeine intake and observe how your body reacts.
- Consider opting for decaffeinated versions of your favorite beverages.

- Stay hydrated with water as the primary beverage.

Limiting Fat Intake and Making Healthy Fat Choices

Now, let's navigate the delicate balance of managing fat intake. Too much fat is like throwing fuel on the inflammation fire, but the right kinds of fats are essential for overall health.

1. Limiting Saturated and Trans Fats: Saturated fats and trans fats are like the villains in the fat world. Found in fried foods, processed snacks, and certain animal products, these fats can contribute to inflammation and are best kept to a minimum in a pancreatitis-friendly diet.

Tips:

- Read food labels to identify and avoid products high in saturated and trans fats.

- Opt for lean cuts of meat and choose cooking methods like grilling or baking instead of frying.

2. Choosing Healthy Fats: Healthy fats are like the superheroes in the fat world. They play a crucial role in various bodily functions and can even have anti-inflammatory properties.

- **Monounsaturated Fats:** Found in olive oil, avocados, and nuts, these fats can be included in moderation.
- **Polyunsaturated Fats:** Found in fatty fish, flaxseeds, and walnuts, these fats, especially omega-3 fatty acids, have anti-inflammatory benefits.

Tips:

- Use olive oil as a primary cooking oil.
- Include fatty fish like salmon or mackerel in your diet a couple of times a week.

- Snack on a handful of nuts for a healthy dose of monounsaturated fats.

3. Portion Control for Fats: Even healthy fats should be consumed in moderation. Portion control is like the golden rule to prevent overwhelming your digestive system.

Tips:

- Measure cooking oils instead of free-pouring.
- Be mindful of serving sizes for nuts and seeds.

CHAPTER 6

Meal Timing and Portion Control

Welcome to the rhythmic dance of mealtime – where timing and portion control take center stage in supporting your pancreas on its journey to health. In this chapter, we'll explore the importance of regular, small meals, strategies for portion control that feel intuitive rather than restrictive, and practical tips for managing meals throughout the day.

Importance of Regular, Small Meals

Imagine your digestive system as a finely tuned orchestra, and each meal is a note contributing to the harmonious melody. The importance of regular, small meals lies in creating a steady rhythm that supports your pancreas and digestive system. Here's why it matters:

1. Avoiding Overwhelm: Large meals can be like an unexpected flood for your digestive system, overwhelming your pancreas with a sudden influx of food. By breaking your daily intake into smaller, more frequent meals, you allow your pancreas to handle manageable portions, preventing stress and potential inflammation.

2. Stabilizing Blood Sugar: Regular meals spaced throughout the day help maintain stable blood sugar levels. This is particularly crucial for individuals with pancreatitis, as blood sugar spikes and crashes can contribute to discomfort and strain on the pancreas. Think of it as providing a steady stream of fuel to keep your metabolic engine running smoothly.

3. Supporting Digestion: Digestion is a continuous process, and small, regular meals keep the digestive system engaged without exhausting it. It's like feeding your digestive orchestra a steady stream of sheet music, ensuring that they can play without missing a beat.

4. Preventing Hunger Pangs: Regular meals help prevent intense hunger pangs. When you let yourself get too hungry, you're more likely to make poor food choices or overeat. Small, balanced meals throughout the day keep hunger at bay, allowing you to make mindful choices and maintain control over your diet.

Strategies for Portion Control

Now that we understand the importance of regular, small meals, let's explore practical strategies for portion control – the art of balancing the quantity of food you eat without feeling deprived.

1. Use Smaller Plates: The size of your plate can influence your perception of portion sizes. Using smaller plates tricks your mind into thinking you have a full plate, even with smaller portions. It's like a visual illusion that helps with portion control without feeling like you're cutting back.

2. Be Mindful of Serving Sizes: Familiarize yourself with standard serving sizes for different food groups. This awareness can guide you in preparing and consuming meals with appropriate portions. It's like having a mental measuring tape for your plate.

3. Listen to Your Body: Your body is an excellent guide when it comes to portion control. Pay attention to hunger and fullness cues. Eat slowly and savor each bite, allowing your body the time it needs to signal when it's satisfied. It's like having an internal portion control mechanism.

4. Pre-portion Snacks: Instead of snacking directly from a larger package, pre-portion snacks into smaller containers or bags. This prevents mindless eating and encourages awareness of portion sizes. It's like having a snack plan that aligns with your overall portion control goals.

5. Practice the 80/20 Rule: Aim to fill your plate with 80% nutrient-dense foods (fruits, vegetables, lean proteins) and leave 20% for indulgences. This way, you can enjoy your favorite treats without overdoing it. It's like finding a balance between nourishment and enjoyment.

Tips for Managing Meals Throughout the Day

Now, let's explore practical tips for managing meals throughout the day – from breakfast to dinner and all the snacks in between.

1. Eat Breakfast: Breakfast is the jumpstart your body needs after a night of fasting. Aim for a balanced meal that includes proteins, whole grains, and fruits or vegetables. It's like giving your digestive system a wake-up call and setting a positive tone for the day.

2. Plan Snacks: Incorporate planned snacks into your day to prevent extreme hunger between meals. Opt for nutrient-dense snacks like a piece of fruit, a handful of nuts, or yogurt. It's like providing your body with mini refueling stations throughout the day.

3. Hydrate Between Meals: Sometimes, feelings of hunger can be confused with dehydration. Stay hydrated between meals by drinking water or herbal teas. It's like giving your body the refreshment it needs without reaching for unnecessary snacks.

4. Include Protein in Every Meal: Protein helps keep you feeling satisfied and supports muscle repair. Include a source of protein in each meal, whether it's lean meat, tofu, beans, or yogurt. It's like the anchor that keeps your meal steady and fulfilling.

5. Mindful Eating: Practice mindful eating by being present during meals. Avoid distractions like phones or TV and savor each bite. This helps you recognize when you're full and prevents overeating. It's like creating a dining experience that nourishes both your body and soul.

6. Evening Meals: Plan your evening meals to be lighter and easier to digest. This can help prevent discomfort before bedtime. It's like winding down the digestive orchestra, allowing it to rest peacefully through the night.

CHAPTER 7

Lifestyle Factors for Pancreatitis Management

Welcome to the holistic realm of pancreatitis management, where lifestyle factors play a crucial role in supporting your pancreas on its journey to health. In this chapter, we'll explore the significance of incorporating physical activity for overall well-being, stress management techniques that act as soothing balms for both body and mind, and the fundamental importance of staying hydrated in nurturing your pancreas.

Incorporating Physical Activity for Overall Health:

Picture your body as a finely tuned machine, and physical activity as the oil that keeps the gears running smoothly. When it comes to managing pancreatitis, incorporating regular exercise is not just about burning calories – it's about supporting your overall health and aiding the healing process. Let's explore why physical activity is a key player in the pancreatitis management symphony:

1. Enhancing Digestive Function: Exercise is like a gentle massage for your internal organs, including the pancreas. It stimulates blood flow and enhances digestive function, helping your pancreas perform its duties more efficiently. It's akin to a supportive hand guiding your digestive orchestra to a harmonious melody.

2. Managing Weight: Maintaining a healthy weight is crucial for pancreatitis management. Excess weight can strain your pancreas and contribute to inflammation. Regular physical activity, whether it's walking, swimming, or gentle yoga, helps manage weight and reduces the burden on your pancreas. It's like giving your pancreas a break from carrying unnecessary baggage.

3. Improving Insulin Sensitivity: Physical activity has a positive impact on insulin sensitivity. This is particularly important for individuals with pancreatitis, as it helps regulate blood sugar levels. It's like fine-tuning the communication between insulin and your cells, ensuring a smooth process of energy utilization.

4. Boosting Mood and Energy Levels: Exercise releases endorphins, the feel-good hormones that act as natural mood lifters. When managing a health condition like pancreatitis, maintaining a positive mindset is crucial. Additionally, regular physical activity boosts energy levels, helping you navigate daily tasks with more vitality. It's like infusing your body with a dose of natural joy and vigor.

5. Supporting Cardiovascular Health: Pancreatitis can be linked to cardiovascular issues, and exercise plays a key role in maintaining heart health. Activities like brisk walking, jogging, or cycling promote cardiovascular fitness, reducing the risk of associated complications. It's like giving your heart a workout, ensuring it stays strong and resilient.

6. Strengthening Muscles and Bones: Incorporating resistance training into your exercise routine helps strengthen muscles and bones. This is particularly important for individuals with pancreatitis, as it contributes to overall physical resilience. It's like building a sturdy foundation for your body to withstand the challenges it may face.

Tips for Incorporating Physical Activity

Now that we understand the importance of physical activity, let's explore practical tips for incorporating it into your daily routine:

1. Start Slow: If you're new to exercise or have been inactive for a while, start slow. Begin with activities like walking or gentle stretching and gradually increase intensity. It's like allowing your body to adapt to the rhythm of movement.

2. Find Activities You Enjoy: Exercise doesn't have to be a chore. Find activities you enjoy, whether it's dancing, gardening, or playing a sport. When you look forward to your workout, it becomes a joyful part of your routine. It's like turning physical activity into a pleasurable hobby.

3. Schedule Regular Breaks: If you have a sedentary job, schedule regular breaks to stretch and move around. Even short bursts of activity throughout the day can make a significant difference. It's like adding musical interludes to break the monotony of stillness.

4. Involve Friends or Family: Exercise can be more enjoyable when shared with others. Involve friends or family members in your activities, whether it's a walking buddy or a workout partner.

It's like turning exercise into a social affair, fostering connection and motivation.

5. Listen to Your Body: Pay attention to how your body responds to different types of exercise. If something causes discomfort or exacerbates symptoms, modify your routine accordingly. It's like having a dialogue with your body, ensuring that exercise is a source of nourishment rather than stress.

Stress Management Techniques

Stress is like a storm that can disrupt the calm waters of your health. When managing pancreatitis, adopting stress management techniques is not just a luxury – it's a necessity. Let's explore why stress management is crucial and practical techniques to integrate into your daily life:

1. Impact on Digestive Health: Stress can wreak havoc on your digestive system, affecting the pancreas and exacerbating symptoms of pancreatitis. It's like sending ripples of chaos through the calm waters of your internal balance. By managing stress, you create a serene environment for your digestive orchestra to perform harmoniously.

2. Immune System Support: Chronic stress weakens the immune system, making your body more susceptible to inflammation and infections. For individuals with pancreatitis, whose immune systems may already be compromised, stress management becomes a protective shield. It's like fortifying your body against potential threats.

3. Emotional Well-Being: Managing a health condition like pancreatitis can be emotionally challenging. Stress management techniques contribute to emotional well-being, providing tools to navigate the ups and downs of the journey. It's like nurturing the emotional garden of your mind.

4. Techniques for Stress Management:

a. Deep Breathing:

- Practice deep breathing exercises to activate the relaxation response. Inhale slowly through your nose, hold for a few seconds, and exhale through your mouth. It's like providing your body with a calming breeze.

b. Meditation:

- Incorporate meditation into your daily routine. Whether it's mindfulness meditation, guided imagery, or mantra meditation, find a practice that resonates with you. It's like creating a peaceful sanctuary for your mind.

c. Progressive Muscle Relaxation:

- Progressive muscle relaxation involves tensing and then slowly releasing different muscle groups. It helps release physical tension and promotes relaxation. It's like a gentle massage for your body and mind.

d. Yoga:

- Yoga combines physical postures with breath control and meditation. It's a holistic practice that promotes both physical and mental well-being. It's like a dance of harmony between body and spirit.

e. Engage in Hobbies:

- Dedicate time to activities you enjoy, whether it's reading, painting, or listening to music. Engaging in hobbies provides an outlet for stress and a source of joy. It's like nourishing your soul with moments of pleasure.

Importance of Staying Hydrated

Water is like the elixir of life for your body, and staying hydrated is fundamental for pancreatitis management. Let's explore why hydration matters and how it contributes to overall well-being:

1. Digestive Support: Adequate hydration is essential for the digestive process. Water helps break down food, making it easier for your pancreas to release digestive enzymes and for your body to absorb nutrients. It's like providing a smooth pathway for your digestive orchestra to perform.

2. Prevention of Constipation: Dehydration can lead to constipation, causing discomfort and potentially exacerbating symptoms of pancreatitis. Staying hydrated ensures regular bowel movements, supporting overall digestive health.

It's like maintaining a clear and unobstructed path for waste elimination.

3. Temperature Regulation: Water plays a crucial role in regulating body temperature. This is particularly important for individuals with pancreatitis, as fluctuations in body temperature can impact overall well-being. It's like having a built-in thermostat that keeps your internal environment stable.

4. Kidney Function: Adequate hydration supports kidney function, helping to flush out waste products from the body. This is important for individuals with pancreatitis, as kidney health is interconnected with overall well-being. It's like providing a cleansing stream for your internal waterways.

5. Tips for Staying Hydrated:

a. Carry a Water Bottle:

- Keep a water bottle with you throughout the day, making it easy to sip water regularly. It's like having a hydration companion by your side.

b. Set Reminders:

- If you tend to forget to drink water, set reminders on your phone or use apps that prompt you to hydrate. It's like having a friendly nudge to stay on track.

c. Infuse with Flavor:

- If plain water is unappealing, infuse it with natural flavors. Add slices of citrus fruits, cucumber, or mint to enhance the taste. It's like turning hydration into a refreshing and enjoyable experience.

d. Monitor Urine Color:

- Pay attention to the color of your urine. Clear or light yellow urine is a good indicator of adequate hydration. Dark yellow or amber urine may signal dehydration. It's like having a visual cue for your hydration status.

e. Include Hydrating Foods:

- Incorporate hydrating foods into your diet, such as water-rich fruits and vegetables. Watermelon, cucumber, and oranges are excellent choices. It's like getting a hydration boost from your plate.

CHAPTER 8

Beyond the Diet: Holistic Approaches to Pancreatitis

Welcome to the final chapter of your journey towards pancreatic health. In Chapter 8, we'll explore holistic approaches that go beyond dietary considerations, delving into complementary therapies, the importance of supportive care and follow-up, and long-term strategies for maintaining pancreatic health. As we conclude, we aim to empower you with a comprehensive toolkit for managing pancreatitis with a holistic perspective.

Integrating Complementary Therapies:

Pancreatitis management extends beyond conventional medical interventions, and integrating complementary therapies can offer additional support. These approaches work alongside traditional treatments to enhance overall well-being. Let's explore some complementary therapies that individuals with pancreatitis may consider:

1. Acupuncture: Acupuncture involves the insertion of thin needles into specific points on the body. This traditional Chinese practice aims to balance the flow of energy, or qi, within the body. For individuals with pancreatitis, acupuncture may help alleviate pain, reduce inflammation, and promote overall relaxation.

How it Works:

- Acupuncture is believed to stimulate the release of endorphins, the body's natural painkillers. It may also have anti-inflammatory effects, contributing to a reduction in pancreatitis-related discomfort.

2. Herbal Medicine: Traditional herbal medicine involves the use of plant-based remedies to address various health concerns. Herbal formulations may be recommended to support pancreatic health and reduce inflammation.

Common Herbal Options:

- Turmeric: Known for its anti-inflammatory properties, turmeric may help manage inflammation associated with pancreatitis.
- Slippery Elm: This herb is thought to soothe the digestive tract and may be beneficial for individuals with pancreatitis.

Important Note:

- Before incorporating herbal remedies, it's crucial to consult with a healthcare professional. Some herbs may interact with medications or have contraindications for certain health conditions.

3. Mind-Body Practices: Practices like yoga, tai chi, and mindfulness meditation fall under the umbrella of mind-body techniques. These approaches emphasize the connection between mental and physical well-being, providing tools for stress reduction and emotional balance.

Benefits:

- Mind-body practices can contribute to stress management, which is particularly important for individuals with pancreatitis. The relaxation and mindfulness components may positively impact overall health.

4. Massage Therapy: Massage therapy involves manipulating the body's soft tissues to promote relaxation and alleviate tension. For individuals with pancreatitis, gentle massage techniques may be considered to reduce stress and ease muscle tension.

Potential Benefits:

- Massage therapy can improve circulation, potentially aiding in the delivery of nutrients and oxygen to the pancreas. It may also provide relief from pain and discomfort associated with pancreatitis.

5. Chiropractic Care: Chiropractic care focuses on the musculoskeletal system, particularly the spine. While not a direct treatment for pancreatitis, chiropractic adjustments may contribute to overall well-being and comfort.

Considerations:

- Individuals considering chiropractic care should communicate openly with both their chiropractor and primary healthcare provider. This collaboration ensures that all aspects of care are aligned.

Supportive Care and Follow-Up

Beyond specific treatments, the journey of managing pancreatitis involves ongoing supportive care and regular follow-ups with healthcare providers. Let's explore why this aspect is crucial for long-term well-being:

1. Regular Monitoring: Regular follow-up appointments allow healthcare providers to monitor your pancreatic health, assess the effectiveness of treatments, and make necessary adjustments to your care plan.

Routine Assessments May Include:

- Blood tests to check pancreatic enzyme levels.
- Imaging studies (such as CT scans or MRIs) to evaluate the pancreas and surrounding structures.

- Monitoring for complications or changes in symptoms.

2. Medication Management: For individuals with chronic pancreatitis, medications may be prescribed to manage pain, reduce inflammation, or support digestive processes. Follow-up appointments provide an opportunity to discuss medication effectiveness, potential side effects, and adjustments to the treatment plan.

Common Medications for Pancreatitis:

- Pain relievers: Nonsteroidal anti-inflammatory drugs (NSAIDs) or acetaminophen.
- Pancreatic enzyme supplements: To aid in digestion.
- Medications to manage underlying conditions contributing to pancreatitis.

3. Nutritional Guidance: Nutritional needs may evolve throughout the course of pancreatitis. Follow-up appointments with a dietitian can ensure that your dietary plan aligns with your current health status, helping you make informed choices to support pancreatic health.

Dietary Adjustments May Include:

- Fine-tuning the balance of macronutrients (proteins, fats, and carbohydrates).
- Modifying specific food choices based on individual tolerance.
- Addressing nutrient deficiencies through supplementation.

4. Emotional and Psychological Support: Managing a chronic condition like pancreatitis can take a toll on mental health. Regular check-ins with healthcare providers, psychologists, or support groups can provide emotional support and coping strategies.

Potential Supportive Approaches:

- Cognitive-behavioral therapy (CBT) to address stress and anxiety.
- Participation in support groups to connect with others facing similar challenges.
- Open communication with healthcare providers about emotional well-being.

Long-Term Strategies for Maintaining Pancreatic Health

As you navigate the journey beyond immediate management, adopting long-term strategies becomes essential for maintaining pancreatic health and overall well-being. Let's explore these strategies:

1. Lifestyle Modifications: Embracing a healthy lifestyle is foundational for long-term pancreatic health. This includes maintaining a balanced diet, engaging in regular physical activity, managing stress, and avoiding known triggers.

Key Lifestyle Elements:

- **Regular Exercise:** Incorporate physical activity into your routine, aiming for a mix of aerobic exercise, strength training, and flexibility exercises.
- **Stress Management:** Continue to prioritize stress-reducing practices, such as meditation, yoga, or hobbies that bring joy.
- **Balanced Diet:** Maintain a diet rich in nutrient-dense foods, with a focus on lean proteins, fruits, vegetables, whole grains, and healthy fats.

2. Regular Screening for Complications: Individuals with chronic pancreatitis may be at a higher risk for certain complications, such as diabetes or pancreatic cancer. Regular screenings and awareness of potential symptoms can aid in early detection and intervention.

Monitoring for Complications May Involve:

- Regular blood glucose monitoring for signs of diabetes.
- Imaging studies to assess the pancreas for structural changes.
- Being vigilant about potential symptoms such as unexplained weight loss or changes in bowel habits.

3. Hydration as a Daily Practice: Maintaining adequate hydration is not only crucial during active management but also as a long-term habit. Make a conscious effort to incorporate sufficient water intake into your daily routine.

Hydration Tips:

- Carry a reusable water bottle with you throughout the day.

- Infuse water with natural flavors like citrus fruits or herbs for added appeal.

- Establish a routine of drinking water at specific intervals, even if you don't feel thirsty.

4. Regular Communication with Healthcare Providers: Long-term pancreatic health requires an ongoing partnership with healthcare providers. Regular communication ensures that any changes in symptoms, dietary needs, or lifestyle factors are addressed promptly.

Open Communication Involves:

- Reporting any new or worsening symptoms promptly.

- Discussing changes in dietary tolerance or preferences.

- Collaborating on adjustments to the overall care plan.

5. Embracing a Holistic Approach: Holistic health involves recognizing the interconnectedness of various aspects of well-being. Embrace a holistic approach by considering not only the physical aspects of health but also the emotional, social, and spiritual dimensions.

Holistic Elements Include:

- **Emotional Well-Being:** Prioritize activities that bring joy and fulfillment. Consider practices like mindfulness, gratitude, or creative pursuits.
- **Social Connections:** Foster meaningful relationships and seek support from friends, family, or support groups.
- **Spiritual Wellness:** Explore practices that align with your spiritual beliefs, whether it's prayer, meditation, or nature connection.

In Conclusion:

Chapter 8 has been our exploration of holistic approaches to pancreatitis, transcending the boundaries of immediate dietary concerns. We've delved into the integration of complementary therapies, emphasized the importance of supportive care and regular follow-ups, and outlined long-term strategies for maintaining pancreatic health. As you embark on the journey beyond this guide, remember that your path is unique, and a holistic approach considers all facets of your well-being. Armed with knowledge and a comprehensive toolkit, you're empowered to navigate the ongoing journey towards optimal pancreatic health.

CONCLUSION

As we conclude this comprehensive guide on managing pancreatitis through diet and holistic approaches, it's crucial to emphasize the individual nature of this journey. Pancreatitis is a complex condition that requires a nuanced approach, considering not only dietary choices but also lifestyle factors and complementary therapies. Let's distill the key takeaways:

1. **Understanding Pancreatitis:**
   - Pancreatitis comes in various forms, each with its own causes and symptoms.
   - Recognizing the importance of early diagnosis and seeking professional medical advice is the first step in managing the condition effectively.

2. **Diet as a Foundation:**

- o Building a foundation for pancreatitis management starts with dietary choices.

- o A well-balanced diet, rich in nutrient-dense foods and low in triggers, plays a pivotal role in supporting pancreatic health.

3. **Complementary Therapies:**

- o Integrating complementary therapies, such as acupuncture, herbal medicine, mind-body practices, massage, and chiropractic care, can provide additional support.

- o Always consult with healthcare professionals before incorporating complementary therapies, ensuring they align with your overall care plan.

4. **Supportive Care and Follow-Up:**

- o Regular follow-up appointments and monitoring are essential for adjusting treatment plans and addressing evolving health needs.

- Nutritional guidance, medication management, and emotional support contribute to a holistic care approach.

5. **Long-Term Strategies:**

- Embracing a healthy lifestyle, including regular exercise, stress management, and hydration, forms the bedrock of long-term pancreatic health.

- Regular screenings for potential complications and open communication with healthcare providers contribute to ongoing well-being.

6. **Holistic Approach:**

- Adopting a holistic approach involves recognizing the interconnectedness of physical, emotional, social, and spiritual dimensions of health.

o Embrace practices that bring joy, foster meaningful connections, and align with your spiritual beliefs for a comprehensive well-being strategy.

Remember, this guide serves as a roadmap, but your journey is unique. Personalize your approach, stay connected with healthcare professionals, and listen to your body's signals. Armed with knowledge and a holistic toolkit, you're empowered to navigate the path towards optimal pancreatic health. May your journey be one of resilience, self-discovery, and holistic well-being.